Fabienne Louise Juvêncio Andrade
Roberta Kelly Mendonça dos Santos
Fabio Correia Lima Nepomuceno

OSPITALIZATION OF FRAIL ELDERLY

Fabienne Louise Juvêncio Andrade
Roberta Kelly Mendonça dos Santos
Fabio Correia Lima Nepomuceno

OSPITALIZATION OF FRAIL ELDERLY

A perspective on support networks

ScienciaScripts

Cover image: www.ingimage.com

This book is a translation from the original published under ISBN 978-3-639-68014-0.

Publisher:
Sciencia Scripts
is a trademark of
Dodo Books Indian Ocean Ltd. and OmniScriptum S.R.L publishing group

120 High Road, East Finchley, London, N2 9ED, United Kingdom
Str. Armeneasca 28/1, office 1, Chisinau MD-2012, Republic of Moldova, Europe
Managing Directors: Ieva Konstantinova, Victoria Ursu
info@omniscriptum.com

Printed at: see last page
ISBN: 978-620-8-52784-6

BOOK

Hospitalisation of frail elderly people represents a growing challenge due to population ageing and the increase in comorbidities associated with this age group. Elderly people in frail conditions, characterised by loss of physiological reserves and greater vulnerability to stressors, present high risks during and after hospitalisation, including functional decline, nosocomial infections and increased mortality. Studies show that these patients are more likely to suffer prolonged hospitalisations and frequent readmissions, which contributes to increased healthcare costs and puts a strain on hospital systems.

Social support networks, made up of family, friends and community services, are fundamental to the recovery and quality of life of hospitalised elderly people. The presence of strong social support can reduce the length of hospital stay, ease the transition back home and minimise the risk of readmissions, as well as contributing to emotional well-being and adherence to treatment.

SUMMARY

The hospitalisation of frail elderly people represents a growing challenge due to population ageing and the increase in comorbidities associated with this age group. Elderly people in frail conditions, characterised by loss of physiological reserves and greater vulnerability to stressors, present high risks during and after hospitalisation, including functional decline, nosocomial infections and increased mortality. Studies show that these patients are more likely to suffer prolonged hospitalisations and frequent readmissions, which contributes to increased healthcare costs and puts a strain on hospital systems.

Social support networks, made up of family, friends and community services, are fundamental to the recovery and quality of life of hospitalised elderly people. The presence of strong social support can reduce the length of hospital stay, ease the transition back home and minimise the risk of readmissions, as well as contributing to emotional well-being and adherence to treatment. Effective social support networks help to manage needs such as assistance with activities of daily living, transport to appointments and monitoring of chronic conditions, reducing the burden on health services.

Research indicates that integrated interventions between the hospital and social support sectors promote more favourable outcomes for frail elderly people. Integrative care models, which combine hospitalisation with home and community support, have been shown to be effective in improving prognosis and reducing post-discharge complications. However, implementing these models requires health policies that strengthen cooperation between social support networks and health systems, with a focus on training carers and supporting long-term care services.

Keywords: Ageing. Frail elderly. Social support. Hospitalisation.

CHAPTER 1 - THE PROCESS OF POPULATION AGEING

In the middle of the 20th century, Brazil was going through a period characterised by high mortality, birth and fertility rates. During this period, the Brazilian population underwent its first changes, with a reduction in infant mortality levels and an increase in life expectancy at birth. Greater access for the population to general water and sewage networks, as well as improvements in health care and access to vaccination campaigns contributed decisively to this (ONRAM, 2005; VASCONCELOS; GOMES, 2012). However, at the same time, the birth rate was above 40 births per thousand inhabitants and women had, on average, more than six children. From the 1970s onwards, fertility changed, mainly as women became more educated and entered the labour market, especially in urban areas (PINHEIRO; GALIZA; FONTOURA, 2009; VASCONCELOS; GOMES, 2012).

Thus, the demographic transition was marked by a fall in the mortality rate, which was more pronounced from the 1980s onwards, followed by a fall in the birth rate, causing significant changes in the population's age structure (ONRAM, 2005; VASCONCELOS; GOMES, 2012).

Currently, people aged 60 and over account for 15.7 per cent of the total Brazilian population (INSTITUTO BRASILEIRO DE GEOGRAFIA E ESTATÍSTICA, 2023). Life expectancy in the country is currently 76 years and in 2030 and 2060 it will rise to 78.7 and 81.2 years respectively. The impact of this growth, which could exceed 40 million people in 2030 and 60 million in 2060, will be felt in the economy, the labour market, family relationships and the health system (INSTITUTO BRASILEIRO DE GEOGRAFIA E ESTATÍSTICA, 2023; PICCINI et al., 2006).

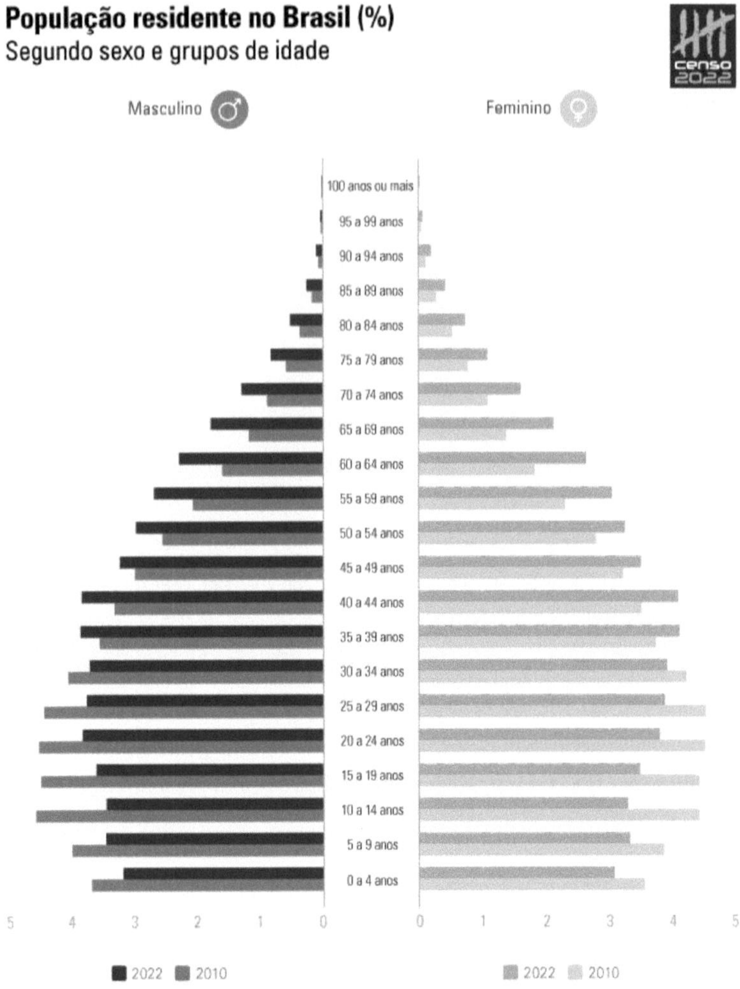

População residente no Brasil (%)
Segundo sexo e grupos de idade

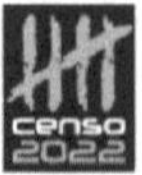

Masculino ♂ Feminino ♀

100 anos ou mais
95 a 99 anos
90 a 94 anos
85 a 89 anos
80 a 84 anos
75 a 79 anos
70 a 74 anos
65 a 69 anos
60 a 64 anos
55 a 59 anos
50 a 54 anos
45 a 49 anos
40 a 44 anos
35 a 39 anos
30 a 34 anos
25 a 29 anos
20 a 24 anos
15 a 19 anos
10 a 14 anos
5 a 9 anos
0 a 4 anos

5 4 3 2 1 0 0 1 2 3 4 5

2022 2010 2022 2010

Figure 1 - Population by age and sex. Source: IBGE, 2023.

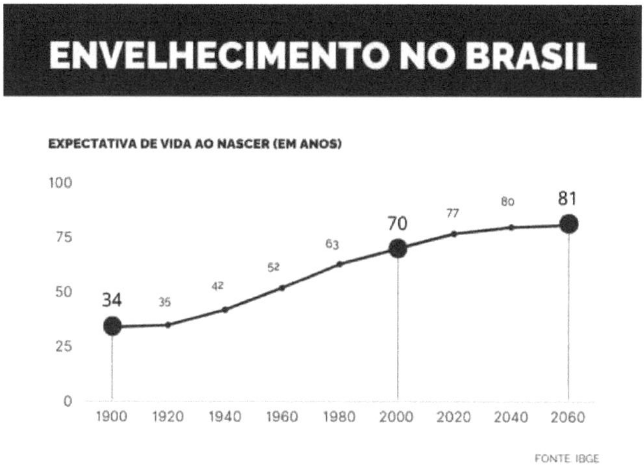

ENVELHECIMENTO NO BRASIL

EXPECTATIVA DE VIDA AO NASCER (EM ANOS)

100
75
50
25
0

34 35 42 52 63 70 77 80 81

1900 1920 1940 1960 1980 2000 2020 2040 2060

FONTE: IBGE

Figure 2 - Estimated and projected life expectancy at birth, by sex (Brazil, 1900-2060). Source: IBGE, 2023.

At the same time as the demographic transition, there was a nutritional transition, characterised by a reduction in the prevalence of nutritional deficits and a significant increase in overweight and obesity. Some factors, such as the rural exodus and industrialisation, as well as the inclusion of women in the labour market, have transformed the quality of food, since meals previously produced by women have given way to industrialised foods, and even meals outside the home. As a result, the prevalence of overweight and obesity has risen considerably and, consequently, chronic non-communicable diseases (CNCDs), mainly diabetes, hypertension, cardiovascular diseases and cancers (SOUZA, 2010). These factors, combined with advances in medicine and technology, have contributed to a change in the epidemiological profile of the elderly in the country (VASCONCELOS; GOMES, 2012).

The epidemiological transition in some European countries and the United States took between one and two centuries, while in Latin America and Brazil it began later and more rapidly, mainly from the 1950s onwards, over a period of 50 years (RAMOS, 2006). This transition has altered the epidemiological panorama regarding the morbidity and mortality of the elderly population, in which infectious and parasitic diseases (IPD), highly prevalent in the young population, have decreased in incidence, while NCDs have increased in prevalence (RAMOS, 2006). However, due to the persistence of diseases associated with poverty and social exclusion, such as tuberculosis and leprosy; the high incidence of malaria; and recurrent dengue epidemics, Brazil has not followed the classic epidemiological transition model, which requires continuous innovation of surveillance models in a diverse and complex social context (DUARTE; BARRETO, 2012).

Thus, even though the substantial improvement in the health parameters of populations observed in the 20th century is far from being distributed equally in different countries and socio-economic contexts, growing old is no longer the privilege of the few (VERAS, 2009).

The ageing process of the Brazilian population is associated with the emergence of more complex and costly chronic diseases, typical of long-lived countries, characterised by chronic and multiple diseases that last for years, requiring constant care, continuous medication and periodic examinations (VERAS, 2009). These complications facilitate the emergence of negative health outcomes such as functional incapacity and, more recently, frailty (GOBBENS et al., 2010).

Figure 3: Rouquayrol; Almeida Filho, 2003.

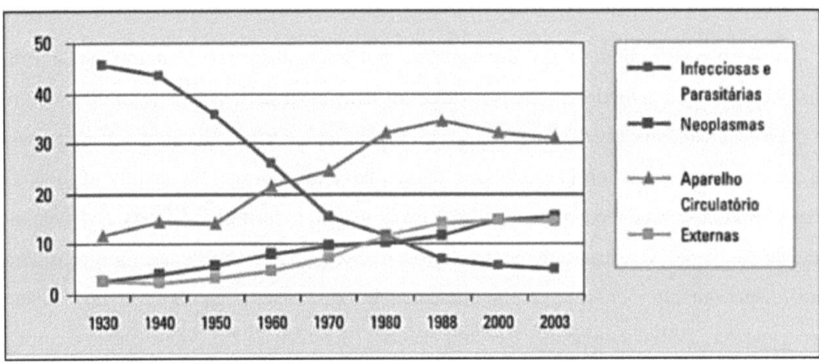

Thus, the ageing of the Brazilian population has presented itself as a major challenge in terms of health and social policies aimed at preserving the health and quality of life of the elderly population (COSTA; FAVÉRO, 2010). The current discourse on policies to care for the elderly envisages a redistribution of activities, providing for the participation of the state, society and the family in actions to protect and assist the elderly. Thus, there is an incentive for the public and private sectors to participate in these policies (SANTOS; SILVA, 2013).

However, the difficulty of public policies to keep up with the rapid growth of the elderly population, which has been recorded in Brazil mainly at the beginning of the 21st century, has resulted in a distortion of responsibilities for dependent elderly people, who end up being taken on by their families as an individual or family problem, due to the absence or precariousness of state support (SANTOS; SILVA, 2013).

CHAPTER 2 - THE FRAIL ELDERLY

The concept of frailty is not new, although there is no consensual definition (FRIED et al., 2001; WOODHOUSE et al., 1988). In this text, frailty is assumed to be a geriatric syndrome, with a cumulative decline in physiological reserves and the ability to maintain homeostasis, which culminates in a state of greater vulnerability (FRIED et al., 2001; RODRÍGUEZ-MAÑAS et al., 2013).

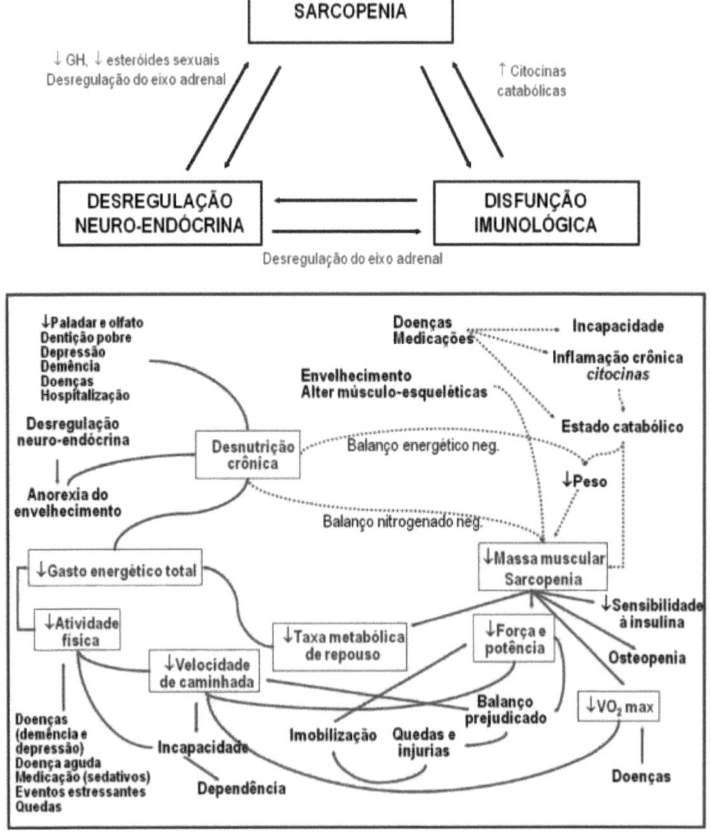

Figure 4 and 5: Predisposing factors for Frailty Syndrome in the Elderly, according to Fried et al. Adapted from Fried et al. 2001.

Frailty began to be debated in the 1970s in developed countries, based on the identification of groups of elderly people who had a combination of morbidities, disabilities and a higher risk of death (GOBBENS et al., 2010). After that time, it was considered synonymous with functional and/or cognitive incapacity (ESPINOZA; HAZUDA, 2008).

Researchers who considered frailty to be a complex interaction of medical and social problems proposed a dynamic model of frailty. They stated that positive factors such as health, functional independence, healthy habits, financial resources and family support interacted with negative factors such as illnesses, particularly chronic ones, physical and cognitive disabilities and the burden on carers, determining whether the elderly were healthy or frail (ROCKWOOD et al., 1994; ROCKWOOD; MACKINIGTH; HOGAN, 2000). If the positive aspects exceeded the negative aspects, the elderly would be healthy. The same authors stated that institutionalised frail elderly people are those who have negative factors outweighing the positive aspects, i.e. those who could not maintain their independence in the community. The frail elderly living in the community, on the other hand, are in a situation where there is a precarious balance between positive and negative aspects (ROCKWOOD et al., 1994, ROCKWOOD; MACKINIGTH; HOGAN, 2000).

Fried et al. (2001), based on the longitudinal *Cardiovascular Health Study* (CHS), identified the frailty phenotype, made up of five indicators: unintentional weight loss, exhaustion, reduced grip strength, reduced walking speed and reduced physical activity.

Fried et al. (2001), based on the longitudinal *Cardiovascular Health Study* (CHS), identified the frailty phenotype, consisting of five indicators: unintentional weight loss, exhaustion, decreased grip strength, decreased gait speed and reduced physical activity. Subsequently, scholars agreed on the importance of a more comprehensive definition of frailty, including mental health and cognition (RODRÍGUEZ-MAÑAS et al., 2013).

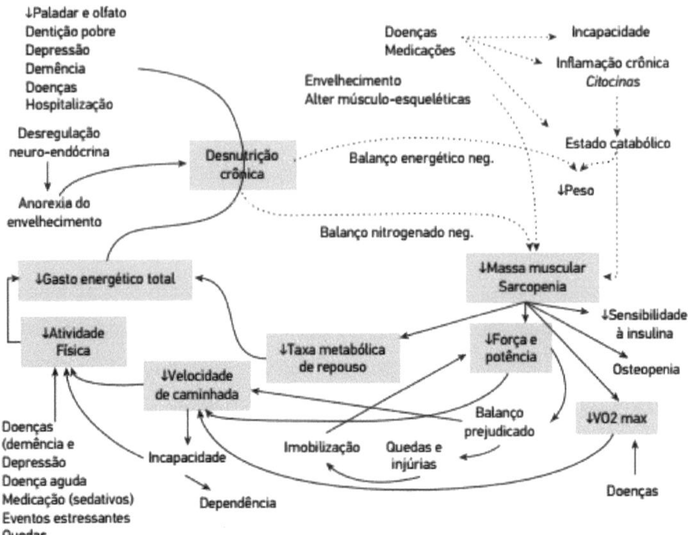

Figure 6: Decreasing energy cycle leading to fragility. Duarte YAO, Lebrão ML. Frailty and ageing (FREITAS et al.2013).

Based on data from Fried et al. (2001), it was estimated that, in a community-dwelling population, 6.9 per cent of the elderly over 65 had the frailty phenotype. Other authors state that between 4.0 and 59.1 per cent of the elderly population are frail.

- Redução da força de preensão palmar
  - abaixo do percentil 20 da população, corrigido por gênero e índice de massa corporal.
- Redução da velocidade de marcha
  - abaixo do percentil 20 da população, em teste de caminhada de 4,6m, corrigido por gênero e estatura.
- Perda de peso não intencional
  - Acima de 4,5 kg referidos ou 5% do peso corporal, se medido, no último ano
- Sensação de exaustão
  - Auto-referida (Questões do questionário CES-D)
- Atividade física baixa
  - Abaixo do percentil 20 da população, em kcal/semana (Minnesota Leisure Time Activity Questionnaire, versão curta)

Chart 1. Frailty criteria, according to Fried et al. The presence of three criteria classifies an elderly person as frail, the presence of one or two as pre-frail and the absence of criteria as non-frail. Adapted from Fried et al. 2001.

With regard to institutionalised elderly people, the prevalence of frailty can be considered high when compared to studies carried out on community-dwelling elderly people, which reported frailty rates of between 19 and 75.6% (KOJIMA, 2015).

Although it is not synonymous with these conditions, frailty syndrome is associated with greater susceptibility to adverse health events, including functional decline, hospitalisation and institutionalisation, thus requiring greater demand on health services at various levels (FRIED et al., 2001; JONES; SONG; ROCKWOOD et al., 2005). Thus, the early identification of frail elderly people allows for interventions that can prevent the occurrence of some diseases, reducing the intensive use and expense of hospital services (GUERRA; RAMOS-CERQUEIRA, 2007).

Similarly, the Brazilian Ministry of Health (MoH), in 2006, through the National Health Policy for the Elderly (PNSPI), considered those who are frail or in a situation of frailty to be frail: is bedridden; has recently been hospitalised for any reason; has diseases causing functional incapacity, such as stroke, dementia syndromes and other neurodegenerative diseases, alcoholism, terminal neoplasia and limb amputations; has at least one basic functional incapacity; lives in situations of domestic violence; or lives in an ILPI (BRASIL, 2006).

In this context, the demand for formal health care for the frail elderly is increasing, and institutionalisation is a frequent outcome for this group (BERGMAN et al., 2007).

CHAPTER 3 - THE SOCIAL SUPPORT NETWORKS OF THE ELDERLY

Social support is still a concept under construction, representing the resources made available by groups and/or people with whom people have systematic contact and which result in positive emotional effects and/or behaviours (SLUZKI, 1997; DUE et al., 1999). This can be of the instrumental or material type, which refers to concrete help such as providing for material needs in general, help with practical jobs (cleaning the house, preparing meals, providing transport) and financial help; affective, which involves expressions of love and affection; emotional, which refers to empathy, affection, love, trust, esteem, affection, listening and interest; and positive social interaction, which refers to the availability of people for fun and relaxation (DUE et al., 1999, OSTERGREN et al., 1991, PINTO at al., 2006).

Social support networks for the elderly can be considered formal and informal. Formal networks are made up of public policies aimed at the elderly population in general, including health care services, legal institutions guaranteeing rights, social security bodies, among others. Informal networks are made up of family, community, friends and neighbours (LEMOS; MEDEIROS, 2002). In addition, each member of the social network can be analysed according to versatility (how many functions the friends perform), reciprocity (whether the individual being assisted also performs an equivalent function), intensity (or commitment to the relationship, defined as the degree of intensity), frequency of contact and history of the relationship (SLUZKI, 1997).

Pagotto et al. (2011), Rosset et al. (2011), Duarte et al. (2005), Lima-Costa et al. (2004) found that 9.4%, 13.2%, 13.1% and 16.5% of the elderly lived alone. According to Cesar et al. (2008) and Tohme et al. (2011), the main determinants of living alone are family and personal income, as well as satisfaction with income.

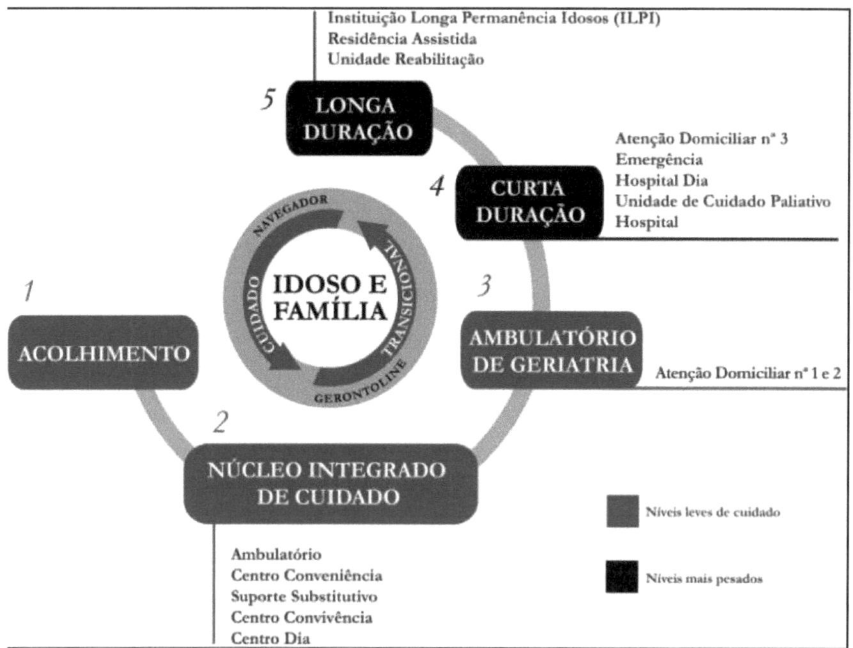

Figure 7: Brazilian model of integrated care for the elderly.

Caption:

Level 1 - Welcome
Level 2 - Integrated Care Centre: Clinical Outpatient Clinic, Day Centre, among other Care facilities.
Level 3 - Geriatric Outpatient Clinic: Home Care complexity 1 and 2
Level 4 - Short-term: Home Care No. 3, Emergency, Hospital, Day Hospital and Palliative Care.
Level - Long-stay: Rehabilitation Unit, Assisted Living Facility and Long-stay Institution for the Elderly (ILPI)

We should consider levels 1 to 3, in grey, to be the light levels, i.e. the lowest cost levels, basically made up of care provided by well-trained health professionals. Efforts should be made to keep patients at these light levels, in order to preserve their quality of life and social participation.

The black areas, the heavy areas, are high cost and are where the hospital and other short and long-stay units are located. Efforts must be made to rehabilitate them and bring them back to the light centres, although this is not always possible.

Therefore, every effort should be made to stay with the elderly person in the first 3 levels of care, in order to maintain their quality of life and reduce costs.

Based on national and international studies, a care model focussed on the elderly and their needs and characteristics was built (OLIVEIRA et al., 2016). The model is structured into five levels, as shown in Figure 7. We should consider, however, that levels 1 to 3 are the soft instances, i.e. lower cost and basically composed of the care of health professionals, all well-trained, and the use of epidemiological screening tools and health monitoring technologies. Efforts must be made to keep patients at these light levels, in order to preserve their quality of life and social participation.

Data from the SABE (LEBRÃO; DUARTE, 2003) and Rede FIBRA (COSTA; CEOLIM; NERI, 2011) surveys found that 57.0% and 52.5% of the elderly population interviewed had a partner. According to Camarano (2006), after separation from their spouse or widowhood, elderly women tend to remain alone. Men, on the other hand, remarry.

Data from the National Social Life, Health, and Aging Project (NSHAP) (CORNWELL et al., 2009), which aimed to study the social relationships of elderly Americans, reported that on average women obtained 61.1 contacts and men 53.4 contacts in order to discuss "important issues". According to Cornwell et al. (2009), the term "important issues" is already well established in social research and prompts the use of names of people heavily accessed by the elderly, where social influence is likely to act.

Fiori et al. (2007) also observed that elderly people living in Berlin had an average of 4.12 (±1.7) regular contacts with family members and 3.14 (±1.9) with friends. A study of French elderly people found that 38.3% of women and 41.0% of men had up to 2 regular contacts (FUHRER et al., 1999). Cornwell et al. (2009) found that 27.7% of the elderly had a low frequency of people to discuss "important matters".

As for the support they actually received, Lebrão and Duarte (2003) observed that 78.0% of the elderly received regular help from services and 20.0% from companions. These authors state that children are also the biggest providers of help, totalling 82.5% from children living in the same household and 39.8% from children living in another household (LEBRÃO; DUARTE, 2003). In another study, Avlund et al (1998) observed that only 25% of women and 7% of men received help with household chores in the month prior to the interview.

Guedea et al. (2006) state that being a support provider contributes significantly to increasing the elderly person's satisfaction with life and to reducing their negative affections. Due et al. (1999) observed that women generally have larger and closer support networks.

However, women do not always enjoy the same health benefits from their social networks as men, since the types of contacts and the help offered by these differ between the genders. While women have more contact with their children and little contact with friends, men generally have the same amount of contact with both (DUE et al., 1999).

A study carried out with older people in Ribeirão Preto (PEDRAZZI, 2008) found higher averages for the size of the network in the various modalities (4.2 for visits; 4.9 for companionship; 3.6 for household chores; 3.2 for personal care; and 3.0 for financial help). This higher frequency found among older people stems from the fact that they have different needs and resources. In addition, older people over the age of 80 are more likely to have lost their spouse and live alone, as well as being in poorer health (ALVARENGA et al., 2011).

Alvarenga et al. (2011) found that 30.6 per cent of those interviewed had a small network for visits; 61.1 per cent for companionship; 78.3 per cent for household chores; 71.4 per cent for personal care; and 54.5 per cent for financial help. Pedrazzi (2008) and Alvarenga et al. (2011) also highlighted the family as the main provider of help.

In view of the above, investigating the social support of the elderly is an important element of a comprehensive protocol for assessing the health of the elderly and can make the difference between the success and failure of an intervention strategy.

To assess the social contact and support received by individuals, there is a graphic instrument called the Minimum Relationship Map, which identifies the relationships that are significant to the individual, delimiting their social support network. This instrument was adapted and modified by Domingues (2000) to identify and characterise the contact and social support network of the elderly. It was then adapted to the demands of this population and named the Minimum Map of Relationships of the Elderly (MMRI).

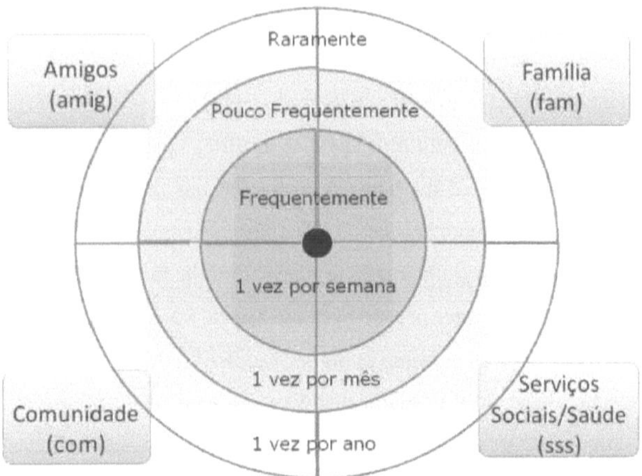

Figure 8 - The Elderly's Minimum Social Relations Map

The MMRI aims to identify the composition and proximity of relationships and the roles played by the components of this network (DOMINGUES, 2000). It is constructed from the answers to five objective questions relating to the daily activities carried out by the elderly person, which are marked on the MMRI in the quadrant that identifies one of the four types of relationship surveyed: friends, family, relations with the community and relations with the health system, and in the circle that denotes the closeness of the relationship, weekly (frequently), monthly (infrequently) and annually (rarely) (Figure 8).

CHAPTER 4 - HOSPITALISATION OF THE ELDERLY

Population ageing, due to the accelerated demographic and epidemiological transition, has led to an increase in demand for health services (LIMA-COSTA; ROUQUAYROL; ALMEIDA FILHO, 2003). The elderly tend to consume more health services, both public and private, and have much higher hospitalisation rates than other age groups, as well as longer hospital stays (AMARAL et al., 2004).

In Brazil, according to the 2013 National Health Survey, of the 200.6 million people living in Brazil, 6.0 per cent were admitted to hospital for 24 hours or more. Of these, hospitalisation of elderly people aged 60 and over was the most prevalent age group, accounting for 10.2% of the total. Of the total number of elderly people hospitalised, 61.8% had their last stay in a SUS hospital (IBGE, 2015).

For the general population, hospitalisations for clinical and surgical treatment were the most frequent. In public healthcare establishments, the proportions were 42.4 per cent and 24.2 per cent, respectively. In private healthcare establishments, the percentages were 29.8 per cent and 41.7 per cent, respectively. The other types of inpatient care had the following proportions for public and private hospitals, respectively: 5.3% and 4.8% for psychiatric treatment; 1.6% and 0.9% for complementary diagnostic tests; and 13.4% and 11.0% for other types of care (IBGE, 2015).

The high prevalence of hospital admissions in the elderly population has been demonstrated by many authors. Dutra et al. (2011) found that 10.1% of elderly Brazilians in the community were hospitalised and 3.3% were readmitted to hospital. Jobim, Souza and Cabrera (2010) found that hospitalisations of the elderly population in two municipalities in the state of Paraná ranged from 25.2 to 31.9% of all hospitalisations. According to Gorzoni and Pires (2006), those aged 60 or over accounted for 20% of SUS hospital admissions in Brazil.

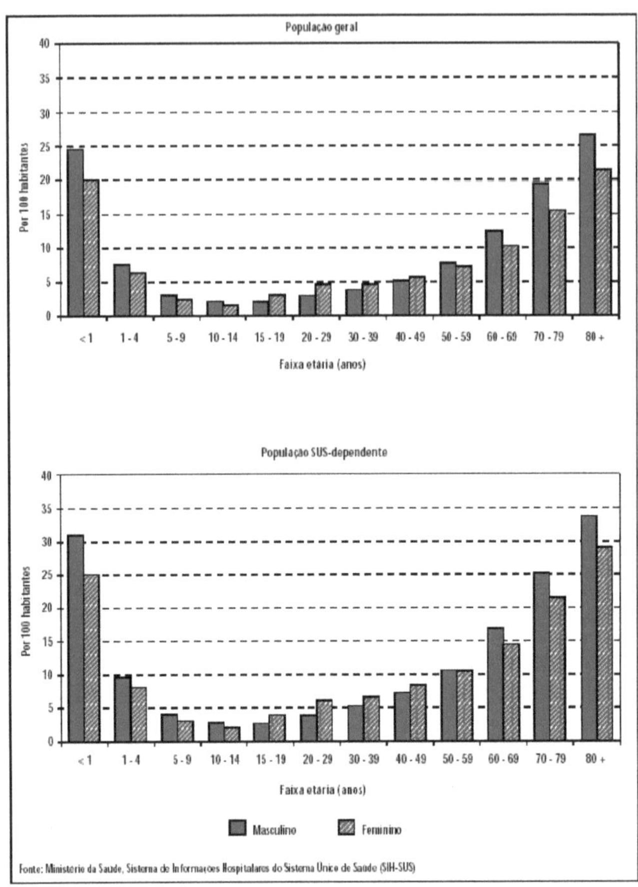

Figure 6 - Hospitalisation rates among the general population and the SUS-dependent population, within the scope of the Unified Health System, 2001.

Studies have shown a significant risk of hospitalisation for frail older adults (AVILA-FUNES et al, 2009; FRIED et al, 2001; KIELY; CUPPLES; LIPSITZ, 2009). Kiely, Cupples and Lipsitz (2009) found that the odds of emergency hospitalisations for frail older adults were 3.4-4.4 higher compared to non-frail older adults.

With regard to elderly people living in LTCFs, Grabowski et al. (2008), in a systematic review, identified hospitalisation rates ranging from 9.0% to 59.0%. Longitudinal studies carried out in the United States found rates of between 11.0% and 25.4% (CARTER; PORRELL, 2003; INTRATOR, ZINN; MOR, 2004; WYSOCKI et al., 2014). A study carried out in Italy found that 11.6 per cent of elderly people were admitted to hospital at least once in a 12-month period (CHERUBINI et al., 2012). In Brazil, researchers from Pelotas-Rio Grande do Sul (RS) found that 23.9% of these elderly people had been hospitalised in a 12-month period (DUCA et al., 2010).

Carter and Porrell (2003) found that the variability in the hospitalisation rate in the United States is related to the type of institution, the qualifications of the nursing staff and the size of the LTCF. Cherubini et al. (2012) also observed that LTCIEs in Italy with a higher number of doctors, nurses, nursing assistants and a higher weekly workload per resident were associated with a lower probability of having their resident hospitalised. According to Duca et al. (2010), the high rate of hospital admissions among institutionalised individuals in Pelotas-Rio Grande do Sul (RS) is due to the higher prevalence of frail elderly people, as well as a high frequency of chronic diseases and disabilities in terms of Basic Activities of Daily Living (BADL). However, Intrator, Castle and Mor (1999) found that there was no significant association between the occurrence of hospitalisation of elderly Americans and the types of facilities in LTCIEs.

The decision to hospitalise an elderly resident of an ILPI is multifactorial and based on elements such as the severity of the illness, the care infrastructure, the wishes of family members and the elderly, as well as financial conditions. This decision requires careful consideration of the risks and benefits of hospitalisation (GORZONI; PIRES, 2006).

Hospitalisation can have a negative impact on the elderly, worsening their health condition, leading to a deterioration in functional capacity and quality of life, which is often irreversible (RIBEIRO et al., 2008). In addition, institutionalised elderly people have an increased risk of iatrogenic complications, which often culminate in worsening health and increased disability (BOOCKVAR et al., 2005; OUSLANDER et al., 2010; PEDONE et al., 2005; WONG, 2010). In some studies, elderly people who were hospitalised had a higher mortality rate than those who were treated in the institution itself (BOOCKVAR et al., 2005; DOSA, 2005).

Therefore, the hospitalisation of institutionalised elderly people, particularly when judged to be potentially avoidable, is considered an indicator of poor quality of care (OUSLANDER; WEINBERG; PHILLIPS, 2000). It has been found that around 9.7% to 60%

of hospitalisations of older people living in LTCIEs were identified as potentially avoidable (GRABOWSKI; O'MALLEY; BARHYDT, 2007; SALIBA et al., 2000; SPECTOR et al., 2013; WYSOCKI et al., 2014).

Young et al. (2010) identified six factors associated with potentially avoidable hospitalisation in institutionalised elderly people: 1- providing training for nursing staff on how to communicate effectively with doctors about a resident's condition; 2- having easy access to laboratory results, preferably in less than 4 hours at weekends; 3- hospital admission being considered by doctors as a last resort; 4- greater adherence to private health insurance; 5- giving preference to the presence of a family member in admissions for acute conditions; 6- having easy access to medical records, laboratory results and electrocardiograms.

There is evidence that implementing strategies and adopting better clinical practice can reduce such hospitalisations (LOEB et al., 2006; OUSLANDER et al., 2009). Furthermore, knowledge of the risk factors associated with hospital admissions can be effective in reducing hospitalisations and healthcare costs, as well as improving the quality of care for the elderly (SPECTOR et al., 2013).

3.1 - Risk factors for hospitalisation of the elderly

In Brazil, the most frequent cause of hospitalisation among the elderly in 2009 was heart failure, which affects 12.1% of women and 14.7% of men, followed by pneumonia (9.1% of women and 10.8% of men), bronchitis (6.5% of women and 10.4% of men) and stroke (5.0% of women and 6.2% of men) are among the six most important causes of hospitalisation for both men and women. Diabetes (4.5%) and Systemic Arterial Hypertension (SAH) (4.2%) are among the six main causes only among women, while inguinal hernia (4.6%) and other ischaemic heart diseases (6.3%) are only among men (IBGE, 2009). In the analysis carried out by Lima-Costa et al. (2000), the main causes of hospitalisation in elderly Brazilians were diseases of the circulatory system, followed by diseases of the respiratory and digestive systems.

Pagotto, Silveira and Velasco (2013), in a study of elderly people in Goiânia-Goiás (GO), found that the main causes of hospitalisation were diseases of the circulatory system (28.4%), infectious and parasitic diseases (9.8%), diseases of the respiratory system (9.8%) and diseases of the digestive system (8.8%). Jobim, Souza and Cabrera (2010) observed that the main causes of hospital admissions among the elderly in Paraná were circulatory and respiratory diseases. This shows that the causes of hospital admissions are concomitant with the disease profile of the elderly population, which is characterised by a predominance of chronic diseases (PAGOTTO; SILVEIRA; VELASCO, 2013).

In a systematic review, researchers pointed out the importance of common geriatric syndromes as predictors of hospitalisation. For these authors, geriatric syndromes are not independent, but there is an overlap between them. Thus, they identified that hospitalisation of the elderly was strongly associated with frailty, functional incapacity and multiple morbidities (WANG et al., 2013). Similarly, Macinko et al. (2011), in a ten-year prospective study in the city of Bambuí - Minas Gerais (MG), also showed the importance of morbidities: each additional chronic condition acquired by the elderly would increase the risk of hospitalisation by up to 27%.

Murray and Laditka (2010), in a one-year cohort study of elderly Americans, identified that polypharmacy, urinary infection and arrhythmias were significantly associated with an increased risk of hospital admission.

Researchers have also identified that hospitalisation of elderly Brazilians was significantly associated with factors related to economic and social issues (economic class A/B had a higher risk compared to classes D and C/E) and health conditions (presence of 5 or more morbidities and unintentional weight loss) (PAGOTTO; SILVEIRA; VELASCO, 2013). It has also been identified that even small differences in social factors, such as additional years of schooling, were important in reducing the risk of hospitalisation among a population of very low socioeconomic status (MACINKO et al., 2011).

Boult et al. (1993), in a four-year cohort study carried out in the United States, identified eight risk factors for high use of hospital services by the elderly: age over 75, male gender, availability of a carer, poor self-perceived health, presence of cardiovascular disease, presence of diabetes mellitus, hospitalisation in the last 12 months and more than six medical consultations in the last 12 months. Based on these factors, researchers in the municipality of Progresso-RS found that elderly people considered to be at high risk suffered 6.5 times more hospitalisations than those classified as low risk (DUTRA et al., 2011).

The results of Buys et al. (2014) showed that community-dwelling elderly people in the United States classified as being at high nutritional risk had a 51.0% increased risk of being hospitalised for general causes over a follow-up of 8.5 years. This increased risk was similar for non-surgical hospitalisations (HR=1.50; 95%CI: 1.11-2.01).

Studies have also investigated the risk factors for hospital admissions in institutionalised elderly people in terms of the intrinsic characteristics of the elderly person and the LTCF. In relation to the elderly, illnesses such as infections, congestive heart failure, circulatory, respiratory and genitourinary system problems were associated with an increased likelihood of being hospitalised (GRABOWSKI et al., 2008). Cherubini et al. (2012) also found that a diagnosis of arrhythmias, urinary tract infection or polypharmacy were associated with a higher risk of being hospitalised. Hutt et al. (2011) found that institutionalised elderly people in hospital had older age, more morbidities and worse functional capacity. However, dementia and terminal illnesses reduced this probability, which may suggest a tendency towards less aggressive treatments for these individuals (GRABOWSKI et al., 2008).

Hwang and Kim (2013) found that the most common signs and symptoms of hospitalisation for institutionalised elderly people were fever (25.8%), followed by pain (11.2%), dyspnea (10.7%), gastrointestinal symptoms (10.4%), falls (9.7%), urinary symptoms (5.2%) and mental changes (5.0%). Most of the participants in this study were older people who were unable to walk or needed help with their Activities of Daily Living (ADLs).

Kruse et al. (2013) found that the main cause of hospitalisation among institutionalised elderly Americans was infection, most commonly pneumonia (33.5%), septicaemia (17.0%) and urinary tract infection (15.4%). Infections were more prevalent in residents with severe ADL impairment. On the other hand, congestive heart failure, hip fracture, kidney failure and stroke were more common in residents with less severe ADL impairment (KRUSE et al., 2013).

In addition, the presence of pressure ulcers has been considered a risk factor for hospitalisation of institutionalised elderly people (CARTER; PORRELL, 2003). The use of feeding tubes and new medications have also been associated with increased long-term hospitalisation (FRIED; MOR, 1997). In addition, previous hospitalisations are positively associated with future hospitalisations (CARTER; PORRELL, 2006).

With regard to LTCIEs, the presence of additional medical resources and greater participation and technical capacity on the part of the doctor have been associated with reductions in hospitalisations (INTRATOR; CASTLE; MOR, 1999). Greater ease in carrying out diagnostic resources, such as x-rays and laboratory tests, can also facilitate the decision to keep the patient in the LTCIE, so that the necessary basic diagnostic investigations can rule out the presence of a serious problem, avoiding unnecessary transfers of the elderly (GRABOWSKI et al., 2008; INTRATOR; CASTLE; MOR, 1999). However, the empirical evidence on these factors is still not well defined (GRABOWSKI et al., 2008).

In view of the above, it has been observed that the hospitalisation of community-dwelling and institutionalised elderly people can occur due to the influence of various factors, including sociodemographic factors, personal habits, health conditions and the organisational characteristics of institutions (GRABOWSKI et al., 2008). Increasing knowledge of these factors can prevent hospitalisation from occurring, as well as improving treatment and patient prognosis (SPECTOR et al., 2013).

3.2 Prognosis and adverse events in hospitalised elderly people

With ageing, individuals tend to reduce their physical activity, which can lead to a reduction in functional capacity (PAULA et al., 2010). According to Siqueira et al. (2004), functional capacity is an important marker of health in hospitalised elderly people. Paula et al. (2010) found that more dependent elderly people stayed in hospital longer, which may suggest that elderly people who are more independent in their ADLs are in better physical condition to recover after being hospitalised. Blanca Gutiérrez et al. (2009) also found an association between physical dependence and length of hospitalisation.

In a study of elderly people admitted to a clinical unit in the municipality of Campos - Rio de Janeiro (RJ), researchers identified a prevalence of 36.6% of hospitalised elderly people in the intermediate care category, followed by 33.3% in minimal care and 26.0% in semi-intensive care (SALES; SANTOS, 2007).

It was also observed, in a Geriatric Inpatient Unit in Rio Grande do Sul, that the elderly who were classified in minimal care had, in their entirety, the outcome as hospital discharge (100.0%). Of the patients in intermediate and semi-intensive care, 9.5% and 40.0%, respectively, died. It was also observed that elderly people aged between 80 and 100 were significantly related to the intermediate and semi-intensive care categories (URBANETTO et al., 2012).

Guerrero and Catalán (2011) observed that the average length of hospitalisation is longer among women, older people over 80, with a high level of dependency and who live alone or in an ILPI. The same authors found a statistically significant association between the duration of hospitalisation and the result of the Pfeiffer Test, i.e. people with severe intellectual deficit had longer hospitalisations, with an average of nine days more than older people with normal cognitive levels (GUERRERO; CATALÁN, 2011).

A study of the morbidity and mortality profile of elderly patients admitted to two hospitals in Rio de Janeiro revealed a death prevalence of 11.7% in the 60-79 age group and 20.3% in those aged 80 or over (AMARAL et al., 2004).

Specifically with regard to institutionalised elderly people, it was identified that the domains most frequently associated with mortality in this population were: diet, physical capacity, shortness of breath and disease diagnosis. These domains provide easily measurable factors that can serve as useful markers for individuals at high risk of mortality (THOMAS; COONEY; FRIED, 2013).

With regard to the term adverse events, it is known that it has currently been used to define unintentional injuries resulting from the intervention of the healthcare team, whether right or wrong, justified or not, but which result in harmful consequences for the patient's health (CARVALHO-FILHO et al., 1998). These can be caused by drug-related use, surgical complication, non-surgical or diagnostic procedures, diagnostic error and hospital-acquired infection (beginning after 48 hours of admission) (SZLEJF, 2010).

The elderly are more susceptible to adverse events due to greater use of the healthcare system, lower functional reserve, more serious illnesses and a greater number of morbidities than young adults. Hospitalisation itself can be a source of functional decline. Medical errors that are well tolerated by young people can be devastating for the elderly (CARVALHO-FILHO et al., 1998).

The prevalence of these events is higher in hospital settings and can range from 3 to 55 per cent of admissions (SZLEJF, 2010). There are few studies of adverse events in Brazil. Mendes et al. (2013), when looking at hospitalised patients in Rio de Janeiro, found an incidence of 7.6% of adverse events, 66.7% of which were preventable . Another study carried out in the Geriatrics Ward of the Hospital das Clínicas at the University of São Paulo Medical School identified a 55% proportion of adverse events, related to longer hospitalisation and in-hospital death (SZLEJF, 2010). The same study found that in-hospital death could be predicted by the occurrence of an adverse medical event, the severity of the illness and functional status at the time of admission (SZLEJF, 2010).

Thus, unnecessary emotional stress and clinical complications resulting from the occurrence of adverse events in hospitalised elderly people increase morbidity and excess healthcare costs. However, these can be prevented, mainly by implementing strategies for better action by the healthcare team, both in decision-making and in access to tests and medical records (YOUNG et al., 2010).

Thus, with the aim of contributing to the qualification of health care in all health establishments, the Ministry of Health, through Ordinance No. 1,377 of 9 July 2013 and Ordinance No. 2,095 of 24 September 2013, approved the basic patient safety protocols: patient identification; pressure ulcer prevention; safety in the prevention, use and administration of medication; safe surgery; hand hygiene practice in health services; and fall prevention (BRASIL, 2013).

Furthermore, improving hospital quality has been widely discussed among hospital institutions, which seek to offer their clients quality care. For this reason, the implementation of management mechanisms aimed at improving quality is essential, especially for the future of the private health sector (GUEDES; LIMA; ASSUNÇÃO, 2005).

CHAPTER 5 - SUPPORT NETWORKS FOR HOSPITALISED ELDERLY PEOPLE

Support networks for hospitalised elderly people are essential components for health promotion and recovery in this population, especially considering the increase in longevity and the prevalence of chronic diseases. This support includes the emotional, social and practical help provided by family, friends, carers and health professionals. Scientific literature shows that robust support networks can improve the adaptation of the elderly to the hospital environment, promote faster recovery and reduce readmission rates and post-discharge complications (CAMARGO et al. 2017).

Studies show that hospitalisation of the elderly can have a significant psychological and emotional impact, intensifying feelings of isolation, anxiety and even depression. The support network, made up of family and friends, helps to reduce these effects by providing a safe and welcoming environment, even outside the family environment. The frequent presence of family members not only provides emotional comfort to the elderly, but also contributes to their engagement with the treatments proposed by the healthcare team, aiding recovery and compliance with care protocols (CAMARGO et al. 2017).

Some specific tools can be used to assess informal support and, consequently, to analyse the network in which the elderly person is inserted. These are important instruments for research and for assessing the health situation for interventions that take into account the various aspects of the elderly person's health, including social aspects. Our aim here is not to delve deeper into understanding these instruments, but we will briefly mention a few so that our readers can find out more about them when the time comes. It is also the understanding of these authors that we need instruments with more careful construction and validation criteria (AERA 2014), and which take into account the specific cultural and social aspects of the Brazilian population. Even so, using the instruments available at the moment can guide professionals towards a less arbitrary assessment and, consequently, more effective management of social support. The table below (table 1) summarises some of the instruments:

Table 2. Instruments for assessing Social Support, year of publication and research approach.

Instrument/Author	Year	Approach
Social support scale for healthy eating habits (PESSINI et al.)	2016	It assessed cross-cultural equivalence and psychometric properties in people aged 24 to 86. The instrument showed cross-cultural equivalence and psychometric properties suitable for application in adults and the elderly.
Minimum Map of Relationships of the Elderly: reproducibility analysis (MMRI) (DOMINGUES)	2000	It presents the reproducibility of the MMRI (cross-cultural adaptation version from 2000 by the same author), which is made up of four quadrants representing family, friends, community and relationships with social or health services. These quadrants are divided into three areas: an inner circle of close relationships, an intermediate circle and another circle of occasional contacts.
Perceived Social Support Scale (EPSS) (Siqueira M.M.M.)	2008	It was applied to people with an average age of 23.93 years. Based on factor analysis, relevant psychometric indices were obtained.
Social support scale for physical activity (Easaf) (REIS et al.)	2011	Evaluates the validity and reliability of the Brazilian version of the social support scale for physical activity in Brazilian adults.
Social Support Scale for People Living with HIV/AIDS (SEIDL; TRÓCCOLI)	2006	The exploratory factor analysis indicated the existence of two first-order factors: emotional social support and instrumental social support.
Social Support Scale of the Pro-Health Study, adapted from the *Social Support Survey of the Medical Outcomes Study* (MOS) (GRIEP et al.)	2005	Composed of items covering five functional dimensions of social support: "material", "affective", "emotional", "information" and "positive social interaction".

Bille-Brahe Social Support Scale (EAS/BB) (GASPARI; BOTEGA)	2002	Questions that assess the individual's level of demand for support and of obtaining help from family and friends.
Social Support and Stress in Childhood and Adolescence Scale (CUPERTINO)	2001	The authors studied the effect of social support in childhood and adolescence on the depressive state of the elderly.
Norbeck Social Support Questionnaire (NSSQ) (ANDRIOLA et al.)	1990	It assesses the multiple sources of social support perceived through three functional components (affection, affirmation and help) and three properties of the subject's social network (number of people in the network, duration of relationships and frequency of contact with network members).

Source: Guedes, MBOG et al. Social support and comprehensive health care for the elderly. Physis: Revista de Saúde Coletiva [online]. 2017, v. 27, n. 04 [Accessed 24 October 2020] , pp. 1185-1204.

Social support is seen as a protective factor, as it promotes the development of resilience and helps the elderly to face the hospitalisation process with more confidence. Studies show that elderly people with a stronger support network have a better chance of recovery and a better quality of life, even after long periods of hospitalisation (BATISTA; TAVARES, 2013; CAMARGO et al. 2017).

The multidisciplinary team is an essential part of the support network. Health professionals such as doctors, nurses, psychologists, physiotherapists and social workers work together to provide comprehensive, humanised care. This holistic approach enables the physical, emotional and social needs of the elderly to be met. Psychological support interventions and educational guidance offered by these professionals are fundamental to preparing the patient and their family for the period of hospitalisation and, subsequently, for discharge and adaptation to the home environment (BATISTA; TAVARES, 2013; SOUZA; SANTOS; NUNES, 2020).

Studies show that elderly people with more effective support networks have lower rates of complications during hospitalisation and recovery. This support reduces the likelihood of hospital readmissions, as the elderly person, feeling welcomed and encouraged, tends to follow medical advice and preventive post-discharge care more rigorously. In addition, trained family members and carers, who receive information and guidance from the healthcare team, are better prepared to deal with the elderly person's needs at home, preventing risk situations that could lead to further hospitalisation (OLIVEIRA; VIEIRA, 2018).

Despite the benefits, there are some challenges in building effective support networks. Many elderly people face limitations in accessing this support due to factors such as geographical distance from family members, lack of financial resources and the absence of public policies that encourage community care. Another challenge lies in the overload of family members, who often accumulate care responsibilities without adequate support (DUARTE; LEBRÃO, 2012).

FINAL CONSIDERATIONS

Support networks for hospitalised elderly people are fundamental to ensuring patient-centred care, promoting emotional well-being, adherence to treatment and more effective recovery. It involves family, friends, carers and health professionals. This network helps maintain the bond with the family and community environment, reducing feelings of isolation and anxiety, which are common during hospitalisation. The emotional support offered by family and friends strengthens the resilience of the elderly, as well as increasing adherence to treatment and the ability to cope with chronic illnesses and debilitating conditions.

Strengthening these networks is essential and requires effective collaboration between family members, health professionals and public policies. Investing in caregiver support programmes, health education actions and community initiatives can be decisive in guaranteeing ageing with quality and dignity for hospitalised elderly people.

REFERENCES

ALVARENGA, M. R. M.; OLIVEIRA, M. A. C.; DOMINGUES, M. A. R.; AMENDOLA, F.; FACCENDA, O. Social support network of the elderly cared for by Family Health teams. **Ciênc Saúde Coletiva**, v. 16, n. 5, p. 2603-2611, 2011.

AMARAL, A. C. S. et al. Morbidity and mortality profile of hospitalised elderly patients. **Cadernos de Saúde Pública**, Rio de Janeiro, v. 20, n. 6, p. 1617-1626, dec. 2004.

AMERICAN EDUCATIONAL RESEARCH ASSOCIATION (AERA). American Psychological Association (APA). National Council on Measurement in Education (NCME). The standards for educational and psychological testing. New York: American Educational Research Association, 2014.

AVILA-FUNES, J. A. et al. Cognitive impairment improves the predictive validity of the pheno-type of frailty for adverse health outcomes: The three-city study. **Journal of the American Geriatrics Society**, New York, v. 57, n. 3, p. 453-461, mar. 2009.

AVLUND, K.; DAMSGAARD, M. T.; HOLSTEIN, B. E. Social relations and mortality. An eleven year follow-up study of 70-year-old men and women in Denmark. **Soc Sci Med.**, v. 47, n. 5, p. 635-643, 1198.

BATISTA, P. S.; TAVARES, D. M. S. Social support network of elderly people hospitalised in a public hospital. **Ciência & Saúde Coletiva**, v. 18, n. 12, 3453-3462, 2013.

BERGMAN, H.; FERRUCCI, L.; GURALNIK, J.; HOGAN, D. B.; HUMMEL, S.; KARUNANANTHAN, S.; WOLFSON, C. Frailty: an emerging research and clinical paradigm-issues and controversies. **The Journals of Gerontology Series A: Biological Sciences and Medical Sciences**, v.62, n.7, p.731-737, 2007.

BLANCA GUTIÉRREZ, J. J. et al. The increase of patient independence in hospital. **Enfermería Global**, Murcia, n. 16, Jun. 2009.

BOOCKVAR, K. S. et al. Outcomes of infections in nursing home residents with and without early hospital transfer. **Journal of the American Geriatrics Society**, New York, v.53, n. 4, p. 590-596, Apr. 2005.

BOULT, C. et al. Screening elders for risk of hospital admission. **Journal of the American Geriatrics Society**, New York, v. 41, n. 8, p. 811-817, Aug. 1993.

BRAZIL. Basic Patient Safety Protocols. **Ordinance n. 2.095, of 24 September 2013**. Brasília, DF: Ministry of Health, 2013.

BUYS, David R. et al. Nutritional risk and body mass index predict hospitalisation, nursing home admissions, and mortality in community-dwelling older adults: results from the UAB Study of Aging with 8.5 years of follow-up. **The Journals of Gerontology Series A: Biological Sciences and Medical Sciences,** North Carolina, v. 69, n. 9, p. 1146-1153, Sep. 2014.

CAMARANO, A. A. Ageing of the Brazilian population: a demographic contribution. In: Freitas EV, Cançado FAX, Gorzoni ML (Org). **Treatise on geriatrics and gerontology**. 2.ed. Rio de Janeiro: Guanabara Koogan; 2006.

CAMARGOS, M. C. S.; DIAS, R. C.; DIAS, J. M. D.; FREIRE, M. T. A. Quality of life and social support network in hospitalised elderly people. **Revista Brasileira de Geriatria e Gerontologia**, v. 20, n.3, 310-319, 2017.

CARTER, Mary W.; PORELL, Frank W. Variations in hospitalisation rates among nursing home residents: The role of facility and market attributes. **Gerontologist**, Washington, v. 43, n. 2, p. 175-191, aug. 2003.

CARVALHO-FILHO, E. T. et al. Iatrogenesis in hospitalised elderly patients. **Revista Saúde Pública**, São Paulo, v. 32, n. 1, p. 36-42, feb. 1998.

CESAR, J. A.; OLIVEIRA-FILHO, J. A.; BESS, G.; CEGIELKA, R.; MACHADO, J.; GONÇALVES, T. S. et al. Profile of elderly residents in two poor municipalities in the North and Northeast regions of Brazil: results of a population-based cross-sectional study. **Cad Saúde Pública**, v. 24, n. 8, p. 1835-1845, 2008.

CHERUBINI, Antonio et al. Predictors of hospitalisation in Italian nursing home residents: the U.L.I.S.S.E. project. **Journal of the American Medical Directors Association**, Washington, v. 13, n. 1, p. 84.e5-84.e10, jan. 2012.

CORNWELL, B.; SCHUMM, L. P.; LAUMANN EO, G. J. Social Networks in the NSHAP Study: Rationale, Measurement, and Preliminary Findings. **J Gerontol B Psychol Sci Soc Sci**, v. 64B, suppl1, p. i47-i55, 2009.

COSTA, S. V.; CEOLIM, M. F.; NERI, A. L. Sleep problems and social support: a multicentre study of frailty in elderly Brazilians. **Rev Latino-Am Enfermagem**, v. 19, n. 4, p. 920-927, 2011.

COSTA, F. G.; FAVÉRO, M. H. The transformation of social representations of ageing: an intervention proposal. **Fragmentos de Cultura**, Goiânia, v. 20, n. 5/6, p. 255-266, May/June 2010.

DOMINGUES, M. A. R. C. **Mapa Mínimo de Relações: adaptation of a graphic instrument for configuring the social support network of the elderly**. São Paulo. Thesis [Doctorate in Public Health] - University of São Paulo; 2004.

DOSA, D. Should I hospitalise my resident with nursing home-acquired pneumonia? J **Journal of the American Medical Directors Association**, Washington, v. 6, n. 5, p. 327-333, Sep/Oct 2005.

DUARTE, E. C.; BARRETO, S. M. Demographic and epidemiological transition: Epidemiology and Health Services revisits and updates the theme. **Epidemiologia e Serviços de Saúde**, Brasília, v. 21, n. 4, p. 529-532, dec. 2012.

DUARTE, Y. A. O.; LEBRÃO, M. L. **Assistance to the elderly**: conceptual and methodological aspects in public health. São Paulo: Atheneu, 2012.

DUARTE, Y. A. O.; LEBRÃO, M. L.; LIMA, F. D. Contribution of household arrangements to meeting the care demands of the functionally impaired elderly in São Paulo, Brazil. **Rev Panam Salud Pública**, v. 17, n. 5/6, p. 370-378, 2005.

DUCA, G. F. D. et al. Hospitalisation and associated factors among residents of long-term care institutions for the elderly. **Cadernos de Saúde Pública**, Rio de Janeiro, v. 26, n. 7, p. 1403-1410, jul. 2010.

DUE, P.; HOLSTEIN, B.; LUND, R.; MODVIG, J.; AVLUND, K. Social relations: Network, support and relational strain. **Social Science & Medicine**, v. 48, n. 5, p. 661-673, 1999.

DUTRA, M. M. et al. Predictive validity of an instrument for identifying elderly people at risk of hospitalisation. **Revista de Saúde Pública**, São Paulo, v. 45, n. 1, p. 106-112, feb. 2011.

ESPINOZA, S. E.; HAZUDA, H. P. Frailty in older Mexican-American and European-American adults: is there an ethnic disparity? **Journal of the American Geriatrics Society**, New York, v. 56, n. 9, p. 1744-1749, sep. 2008.

FIORI, K. L.; SMITH, J.; ANTONUCCI, T. C. Social Network Types Among Older Adults: A Multidimensional Approach. J **Gerontol B Psychol Sci Soc Sci**, v. 62, n. 6, p. P322-P330, 2007.

FREITAS, E. V.; PY, L.; CANÇADO, F. A. X.; DOLL, J.; GORZONI, M. L. Tratado de geriatria e gerontologia. 3. ed. Rio de Janeiro: Guanabara Koogan, 2013.

FRIED, T. R.; MOR, V. Frailty and hospitalisation of long-term stay nursing home residents. **Journal of the American Geriatrics Society**, New York, v. 45, n. 3, p. 265-269, mar. 1997.

FRIED, L. P.; TANGEN, C. M.; WALSTON, J.; NEWMAN, A. B.; HIRSCH, C.; GOTTDIENER, J.; SEEMAN, T.; TRACY, R.; KOP, W. J.; BURKE, G.; MCBURNIE, M. A. Frailty in older adults: evidence for a phenotype. **Journal of Gerontology,** v.56, n.3, p M146-M156, 2001.

FUHRER, R.; DUFOUIL, C.; ANTONUCCI, T. C.; SHIPLEY, M. J.; HELMER, C.; DARTIGUES, J. F. Psychological disorder and mortality in French older adults: do social relations modify the association? **Am J Epidemiol**, v. 149, n. 2, p. 116-126, 1999.

GOBBENS, R. J. J. et al. Determinants of Frailty. **Journal of the American Medical Directors Association**, Washington, v. 11, n. 5, p. 356-364, jun. 2010.

GORZONI, M. L.; PIRES, S. L. Elderly patients in general hospitals. **Revista de Saúde Pública**, São Paulo, v. 40, n. 6, p. 1124-1130, dec. 2006.

GRABOWSKI, D. C.; O'MALLEY, A. James; BARHYDT, Nancy R. The costs and potential savings associated with nursing home hospitalisations. **Health Aff (Millwood)**, Washington, v.

26, n. 6, p. 1753-1761, Nov./Dec. 2007.

GRABOWSKI, D. C. et al. Predictors of nursing home hospitalisation. A review of the literature. **Medical Care Research and Review**, New York, v. 65, n. 1, p.3-39, feb. 2008.

GUEDEA, M. T. D.; ALBUQUERQUE, F. J. B.; TRÓCCOLI, B. T.; NORIEGA, J. A. V.; SEABRA, M. A. B.; GUEDEA, R. L. D. Relationship between subjective well-being, coping strategies and social support in the elderly. **Psychol Reflex Crit**, v. 19, n. 2, p. 301-308, 2006.

GUEDES, R. M. A.; LIMA, F. P. A.; ASSUNCAO, A. Á. The quality programme in the hospital sector and real nursing activities: the case of medication. **Ciência & Saúde Coletiva**, Rio de Janeiro, v. 10, n. 4, p. 1063-1074, dec. 2005.

GUEDES, M. B. O. G. et al. Social support and comprehensive health care for the elderly. Physis: Revista de Saúde Coletiva [online]. v. 27, n. 04, pp. 1185-1204 , 2017.

GUERRA, I. C.; RAMOS-CERQUEIRA, A. T. A. Risk of repeated hospitalisations in elderly users of a school health centre. **Cadernos de Saúde Pública**, Rio de Janeiro, v. 23, n. 3, p. 585-592, mar. 2007.

GUERRERO, L. L.; CATALÁN, A. G. Biopsychosocial variables related to the duration of hospitalisation in the elderly. **Revista Latino-Americana de Enfermagem**, Ribeirão Preto, v. 19, n. 6, 08 telas, nov./dez. 2011.

HUTT, E. et al. Regional variation in mortality and subsequent hospitalisation of nursing residents with heart failure. **Journal of the American Medical Directors Association**, Washington, v. 12, n. 8, p. 595-601, Oct. 2011.

HWANG, J. H.; KIM, S. H. Seasonal variations in acute hospitalisation and mortality among nursing home residents: Results from LOVE (Long-term care of Old people Via KorEan Nursing Home Network) study. **European Geriatric Medicine,** Vienna, v. 4, n. 3, p. 172-175, jun. 2013.

BRAZILIAN INSTITUTE OF GEOGRAPHY AND STATISTICS. **Sociodemographic and Health Indicators in Brazil.** Rio de Janeiro, 2009.

BRAZILIAN INSTITUTE OF GEOGRAPHY AND STATISTICS. **National health survey 2013**: access to and use of health services, accidents and violence. Rio de Janeiro, 2015.

BRAZILIAN INSTITUTE OF GEOGRAPHY AND STATISTICS. **Projection of the Population of Brazil by Sex and Age**: 2000-2060. Rio de Janeiro, 2023.

INTRATOR, O.; CASTLE, N. G.; MOR, V. Facility characteristics associated with hospitalisation of nursing home residents: Results of a national study. **Medical care**, Massachusetts, v. 37, n. 3, p. 228-237, mar. 1999.

INTRATOR, O.; ZINN, J.; MOR, V. Nursing home characteristics and potentially preventable hospitalizations of long-stay residents. **Journal of the American Geriatrics Society**, New

York, v. 52, n. 10, p. 1730-1736, sep. 2004.

JOBIM, E. F. C.; SOUZA, V. O.; CABRERA, M. A. S. Causes of hospitalisation of elderly people in two general hospitals under the Unified Health System (SUS). **Acta Scientiarum. Health Sciences,** Maringá, v. 32, n. 1, p. 79-83, 2010.

JONES, D. M.; SONG, X.; ROCKWOOD, K. Operationalising a frailty index from a standardized comprehensive geriatric assessment. **Journal of the American Geriatrics Society**, New York, v. 52, n. 11, p. 1929-1933, nov. 2004.

KIELY, Dan K.; CUPPLES, L. Adrienne; LIPSITZ, Lewis A. Validation and comparison of two frailty indexes: The MOBILIZE Boston Study. **Journal of the American Geriatrics Society**, New York, v. 57, n. 9, p. 1532-1539, sep. 2009.

KRUSE, R. L. et al. Activities of Daily Living (ADL) Trajectories Surrounding Acute Hospitalisation of Long-stay Nursing Home Residents. **Journal of the American Geriatrics Society**, New York, v. 61, n. 11, p. 1909-1918, Oct. 2013.

LEMOS, N.; MEDEIROS, S. L. Social support for the dependent elderly. In: FREITAS, E. V.; CANÇADO, F. A. X.; GORZONI, M. L. (Org). **Treatise on geriatrics and gerontology**. Rio de Janeiro: Guanabara Koogan; 2002.

LIMA-COSTA, M. F. F. et al. Health diagnosis of the Brazilian elderly population: a study of mortality and public hospital admissions. **Informe Epidemiológico do Sus**, Brasília, v. 9, n. 1, p. 43-50, Mar. 2000.

LIMA-COSTA, M. F.; FIRMO, J. O. A.; UCHÔA, E. The structure of self-rated health among the elderly: Bambuí project. **Rev Saúde Pública**, v. 38, n. 6, p. 827-834, 2004.

LIMA-COSTA, M. F. F.; ROUQUAYROL, M. Z.; ALMEIDA FILHO, N. Epidemiology of ageing in Brazil. In: ROUQUAYROL, M. Z.; ALMEIDA FILHO, N. (Org.). **Epidemiologia & Saúde**. 6. ed. Rio de Janeiro: Medsi, p. 499-514, 2003.

LOEB, M. et al. Effect of a clinical pathway to reduce hospitalisations in nursing home residents with pneumonia: A randomized controlled trial. **Journal of the American Medical Association**, Washington, v. 295, n. 21, p. 2503-2510, jun. 2006.

MACINKO, J. et al. Predictors of 10-year hospital use in a community-dwelling population of Brazilian elderly: the Bambui Cohort Study of Aging. **Cadernos de Saúde Publica**, Rio de Janeiro, v.27, supl. 3, p.S336-S344, 2011.

MENDES, W. et al. Characteristics of preventable adverse events in hospitals in Rio de Janeiro. **Revista da Associação Médica Brasileira**, São Paulo, v. 59, n. 5, p. 421-428, Oct. 2013.

MURRAY, L. M.; LADITKA, S. B. Care transitions by older adults from nursing homes to hospitals: Implications for long-term care practice, geriatrics education, and research. **Journal of the American Medical Directors Association**, Washington, v. 11, n. 4, p. 231-238, May 2010.

OLIVEIRA, M. R.; SILVEIRA, D. P.; NEVES, R.; VERAS, R.; ESTRELLA, K.; ASSALIM, V. M.; ARAUJO, D. V.; GOMES, G. H. G.; LIMA, K. C. **Elderly in supplementary healthcare: an urgency for the health of society and for the sustainability of the sector Rio de Janeiro**: Agência Nacional **de** Saúde Suplementar; 2016.

OLIVEIRA, E. H.; VIEIRA, N. M. The importance of the social support network for the recovery of hospitalised elderly people. **Cadernos de Saúde Pública**, v. 34, n. 5, 2018.

ONRAM, A. R. The epidemiological transition. A theory of the epidemiology of populatuion change. **The milbank memorial fund quartely**, Malden, v. 83, n. 4, p. 731-757, dec. 2005.

OSTERGREN PO, H. B. S.; ISACSSON, S. O.; TEJLER, L. Social network, social support and acute chest complaints among young and middle-aged patients in an emergency department: a case-control study. **Soc Sci Med**, v. 33, n. 3, p. 257-267, 1991.

OUSLANDER, J. G.; WEINBERG, Andrew D.; PHILLIPS, Victoria. Inappropriate hospitalisation of nursing facility residents: A symptom of a sick system of care for frail older people. **Journal of the American Geriatrics Society**, New York, v. 48, n. 2, p. 230-231, feb. 2000.

OUSLANDER, J. G. et al. Reducing potentially avoidable hospitalisations of nursing home residents: Results of a pilot quality improvement project. **Journal of the American Medical Directors Association**, Washington, v.10, n. 9, p. 644-652, 2009.

OUSLANDER, J. G. et al. Potentially avoidable hospitalisations of nursing home residents: Frequency, causes, and costs. **Journal of the American Geriatrics Society**, New York, v. 58, n. 4, p. 627-635, Apr. 2010.

PAGOTTO, V.; NAKATANI, A. Y. K.; SILVEIRA, E. A. Factors associated with poor self-rated health in elderly users of the Unified Health System**. Cad Saúde Pública**, v. 27, n. 8, p. 1593-1602, 2011.

PAGOTTO, V.; SILVEIRA, E. A.; VELASCO, W. D. Profile of hospitalisations and associated factors in elderly SUS users. **Ciência & Saúde Coletiva**, Rio de Janeiro, v. 18, n. 10, p. 3061-3070, Oct. 2013.

PAULA, F. L. et al. Profile of elderly people admitted to public hospitals in Niterói (RJ) due to falls. **Revista Brasileira de Epidemiologia**, São Paulo, v. 13, n. 4, p. 587-595, dec. 2010.

PEDONE, C. et al. Comparison of digitalis-related adverse events in hospitalised men and women in Italy: An observational study. **Clinical Therapeutics**, Amsterdam, v. 27, n. 12, p. 1922-1929, dec. 2005.

PEDRAZZI, E. C. **Household Arrangement and Family Support for the Elderly. Ribeirão Preto**. Dissertation [Master's in Nursing] - University of São Paulo; 2008.

PINHEIRO, L.; GALIZA, M.; FONTOURA, N. New family arrangements, old social gender conventions: parental leave as a public policy to deal with these tensions. **Revista Estudos Feministas**, Florianópolis, v. 17, n. 3, p. 851-859, dec. 2009.

PINTO, J. L. G.; GARCIA, A. C. O.; BOCCHI, S. C.; CARVALHAES, M. A. B. L. Characteristics of the social support offered to elderly people in a rural area assisted by the PSF. **Ciênc Saúde Coletiva**, v.11, n. 3, p. 753-764, 2006.

RAMOS, L. R. Epidemiology of ageing. In: FREITAS, Elisabete Viana de et al (Org.). **Tratado de geriatria e gerontologia**. 2. ed. Rio de Janeiro: Guanabara Koogan, 2006.

RIBEIRO, A. P. et al. The influence of falls on the quality of life of the elderly. **Ciência & Saúde Coletiva**, Rio de Janeiro, v. 13, n. 4, p. 1265-1273, aug. 2008.

ROCKWOOD, Kenneth. et al. Frailty in elderly people: an evolving concept. **Canadian Medical Association Journal**, Canada, v. 150, n. 4, p. 489-495, feb. 1994.

ROCKWOOD, K.; MACKINIGTH, C.; HOGAN, D. B. Conceptualisation and measurement of frailty in elderly people. **Drugs & Aging, v.**17, n.4, p.295-302, 2000.

RODRÍGUEZ-MAÑAS, L. et al. Searching for an Operational Definition of Frailty: A Delphi Method Based Consensus Statement. The Frailty Operative Definition-Consensus Conference Project. **The Journals of Gerontology Series A: Biological Sciences and Medical Sciences**, North Carolina, v. 68, n. 1, p. 62-67, Jan. 2013.

ROSSET, I.; RORIZ-CRUZ, M.; SANTOS, J. L. F.; HAAS, V. J.; FABRÍCIO-WEHBE, S. C. C.; RODRIGUES, R. A. P. Socioeconomic and health differentials between two communities of long-lived elderly. **Rev Saúde Pública**, v. 45, n. 2, p. 391-400, 2011.

SALIBA, Debra et al. Appropriateness of the decision to transfer nursing facility residents to the hospital. **Journal of the American Geriatrics Society**, New York, v. 48, n. 2, p. 154-163, Feb. 2000.

SALES, F. M.; SANTOS, I. Profile of hospitalised elderly and level of dependence on nursing care: identification of needs. **Texto & Contexto - Enfermagem**, Florianópolis, v. 16, n. 3, p. 495-502, sep. 2007.

SANTOS, N. F.; SILVA, M. R. F. Public policies for the elderly: improving quality of life or reprivatising old age. **Revista FSA**, Teresina, v. 10, n. 2, art. 20, pp. 358-371, Apr./Jun. 2013.

SLUZKI, C. The social network in systemic practice: therapeutic alternatives. São Paulo: Casa do Psicólogo; 1997.

SOUZA, E. B. Nutritional transition in Brazil: analysing the main factors. **Cadernos UniFOA, Volta Redonda**, n. 13, p. 49-53, Aug. 2010.

SOUZA, J. P.; SANTOS, A. A.; NUNES, C. M. O papel da família e dos cuidadores no apoio a idosos hospitalizados. **Revista Kairós**, v. 23, n. 2, 175-191, 2020.

SIQUEIRA, A. B. et al. Functional impact of hospitalisation of elderly patients. **Revista de Saúde Pública**, São Paulo, v. 38, n. 5, p. 687-694, Oct. 2004.

SPECTOR, William D. et al. Potentially avoidable hospitalisations for elderly long-stay residents in nursing homes. **Medical Care**, Washington, v. 51, n. 8, p. 673-681, Aug. 2013.

SZLEJF, C. **Adverse medical events in hospitalised elderly:** frequency and risk factors in a geriatric ward. 2010. 90 f. Thesis (Doctorate in Pathology) - Faculty of Medicine, University of São Paulo, São Paulo, 2010.

TOHME, R. A.; YOUNT, K. M.; YASSINE, S.; SHIDEED, O.; SIBAI, A. M. Socioeconomic resources and living arrangements of older adults in Lebanon: who chooses to live alone? **Ageing and Society**, v. 31, n. 1, p. 1-17, 2011.

THOMAS, J. M.; COONEY, L. M.; FRIED, T. R. Systematic review: Health-related characteristics of elderly hospitalised adults and nursing home residents associated with short-term mortality. **Journal of the American Geriatrics Society**, New York, v. 61, n. 6, p. 902-911, jun. 2013.

URBANETTO, J. S. et al. Degree of dependence of hospitalised elderly according to the patient classification system. **Revista Brasileira de Enfermagem**, Brasília, v. 65, n. 6, p. 950-954, dec. 2012.

VASCONCELOS, A. M. N.; GOMES, M. M. F.. Demographic transition: the Brazilian experience. **Epidemiologia e Serviços de Saúde**, Brasília, v. 21, n. 4, p. 539-548, Oct./Dec. 2012.

VERAS, R. Contemporary population ageing: demands, challenges and innovations. **Revista de Saúde Pública**, São Paulo, v. 43, n. 3, p. 548-54, May/June 2009.

WANG, S. et al. Not just specific diseases: systematic review of the association of geriatric syndromes with hospitalisation or nursing home admission. **Archives of Gerontology and Geriatrics**, Amsterdam, v. 57, n. 1, p. 16-26, Jul./Aug. 2013.

WONG, R. Y. Transferring nursing home residents to acute care hospital d to do or not to do, that is the question. **Journal of the American Medical Directors Association**, Washington, v. 11, n. 5, p.304-305, jun. 2010.

WOODHOUSE, Ken W. et al. Who are the Frail Elderly? **Quarterly Journal of Medicine,** Oxford, v.68, n.255, p. 505-506, jul. 1988.

WYSOCKI, A. et al. Hospitalisation of elderly Medicaid long-term care users who transition from nursing homes. **Journal of the American Geriatrics Society**, New York, v. 62, n. 1, p. 71-78. jan. 2014.

YOUNG, Y. et al. Factors associated with potentially preventable hospitalisation in nursing home residents in New York State: a survey of directors of nursing. **Journal of the American Geriatrics Society**, New York, v. 58, n. 5, p. 901-907, May 2010.

CONTENTS

CHAPTER 1 - THE PROCESS OF POPULATION AGEING 3
CHAPTER 2 - THE FRAIL ELDERLY 8
CHAPTER 3 - THE SOCIAL SUPPORT NETWORKS OF THE ELDERLY 12
CHAPTER 4 - HOSPITALISATION OF THE ELDERLY 17
CHAPTER 5 - SUPPORT NETWORKS FOR HOSPITALISED ELDERLY PEOPLE 26

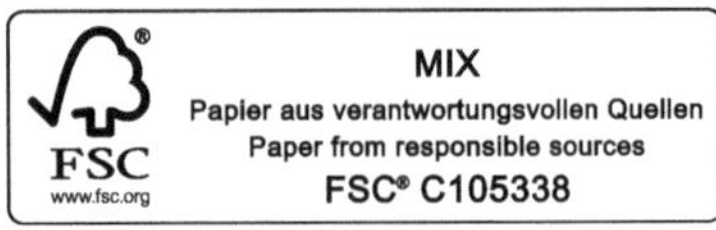

Printed by Books on Demand GmbH, Norderstedt / Germany